MOOD
Journal

This Journal Belongs to:
_____
_____
_____

MOOD & HEALTH TRACKER

Dedication

This Health and Mood Tracker Logbook is dedicated to all the wonderful people who want to practice self-awareness and document their journey.

You are my inspiration for producing this book and I'm honored to be a part of your self-awareness journaling and ongoing routine of balancing your day.

HOW TO USE THIS BOOK

This Mood and Health Tracker book will help guide you through daily documentation of your moods and triggers, and provides prompts for reflections and goal setting. Plus, track food and water intake, doctor appointments, and medical information.

Here are examples of daily tracking, checklists and prompts for you to fill in and keep track of all the details:

1. Fill In - personal Information, emergency contacts and health information

2. Fill in - doctor and medical Information

3. Log - daily emotions, food and water intake and exercise

4. Write down - your daily reflections, positive affirmations and goals

MY INFORMATION

Personal Information

Name: _____
Phone #: _____
Address: _____
Email: _____

Emergency Contact Information

Name: _____
Phone #: _____
Address: _____
Email: _____

Health Conditions

_____
_____
_____
_____

Additional Information

_____
_____
_____
_____

MY INFORMATION

Physician

Name: _____
Phone #: _____
Address: _____
Email: _____

Psychologist/Psychiatrist

Name: _____
Phone #: _____
Address: _____
Email: _____

Nurse/Nurse Practitioner

_____
_____
_____
_____

Pharmacy

_____
_____
_____
_____

Date: _____ Wake-Up Time For Today: _____
Hours Slept Last Night:_____

My Mood:

Morning

Afternoon

Evening

How I Feel Today?
- ❏ Anger/frustration
- ❏ Appetite- increased or decreased
- ❏ Difficulty concentrating/making decisions
- ❏ Energized
- ❏ Happy
- ❏ Hopeful
- ❏ Hopeless
- ❏ Joyful
- ❏ Lack of motivation
- ❏ No energy fatigue/lethargic
- ❏ Sad and/or tearful
- ❏ _____
- ❏ _____
- ❏ _____
- ❏ _____

Exercise
_____
_____
_____
_____

Food & Beverage

Breakfast
_____
_____

Lunch
_____
_____

Supper
_____
_____

Snacks
_____
_____

Water

Positive Things That Happened Today:

_____
_____
_____
_____

Is There Anything I Could Have Done To Improve My Day:

_____
_____
_____
_____

Today, I Am Grateful For:

_____
_____
_____
_____

Positive Affirmations:

_____
_____
_____
_____

Goals/Things I Can Do To Make Tomorrow Better:

_____
_____
_____
_____

Date: _____ Wake-Up Time For Today: _____
Hours Slept Last Night:_____

My Mood:

Morning

Afternoon   **Evening**

How I Feel Today?
- ❑ Anger/frustration
- ❑ Appetite- increased or decreased
- ❑ Difficulty concentrating/making decisions
- ❑ Energized
- ❑ Happy
- ❑ Hopeful
- ❑ Hopeless
- ❑ Joyful
- ❑ Lack of motivation
- ❑ No energy fatigue/lethargic
- ❑ Sad and/or tearful
- ❑ _____
- ❑ _____
- ❑ _____
- ❑ _____

Exercise
_____
_____
_____
_____

Food & Beverage

Breakfast
_____
_____

Lunch
_____
_____

Supper
_____
_____

Snacks
_____
_____

Water

Positive Things That Happened Today:

_____
_____
_____
_____
_____

Is There Anything I Could Have Done To Improve My Day:

_____
_____
_____
_____
_____

Today, I Am Grateful For:

_____
_____
_____
_____
_____

Positive Affirmations:

_____
_____
_____
_____
_____

Goals/Things I Can Do To Make Tomorrow Better:

_____
_____
_____
_____
_____

Date: _____ Wake-Up Time For Today: _____

Hours Slept Last Night: _____

My Mood:

Morning

Afternoon

Evening

How I Feel Today?
- ❑ Anger/frustration
- ❑ Appetite- increased or decreased
- ❑ Difficulty concentrating/making decisions
- ❑ Energized
- ❑ Happy
- ❑ Hopeful
- ❑ Hopeless
- ❑ Joyful
- ❑ Lack of motivation
- ❑ No energy fatigue/lethargic
- ❑ Sad and/or tearful
- ❑ _____
- ❑ _____
- ❑ _____
- ❑ _____

Exercise
_____
_____
_____
_____

Food & Beverage

Breakfast
_____
_____

Lunch
_____
_____

Supper
_____
_____

Snacks
_____
_____

Water

Positive Things That Happened Today:

_____
_____
_____
_____
_____

Is There Anything I Could Have Done To Improve My Day:

_____
_____
_____
_____
_____
_____

Today, I Am Grateful For:

_____
_____
_____
_____
_____
_____

Positive Affirmations:

_____
_____
_____
_____
_____
_____

Goals/Things I Can Do To Make Tomorrow Better:

_____
_____
_____
_____

Date: _____ Wake-Up Time For Today: _____
Hours Slept Last Night:_____

My Mood:

Morning

Afternoon

Evening

How I Feel Today?
- ❏ Anger/frustration
- ❏ Appetite- increased or decreased
- ❏ Difficulty concentrating/making decisions
- ❏ Energized
- ❏ Happy
- ❏ Hopeful
- ❏ Hopeless
- ❏ Joyful
- ❏ Lack of motivation
- ❏ No energy fatigue/lethargic
- ❏ Sad and/or tearful
- ❏ _____
- ❏ _____
- ❏ _____
- ❏ _____

Exercise
_____
_____
_____
_____

Food & Beverage

Breakfast
_____
_____

Lunch
_____
_____

Supper
_____
_____

Snacks
_____
_____

Water

Positive Things That Happened Today:
_____
_____
_____
_____
_____

Is There Anything I Could Have Done To Improve My Day:
_____
_____
_____
_____
_____

Today, I Am Grateful For:
_____
_____
_____
_____
_____

Positive Affirmations:
_____
_____
_____
_____
_____

Goals/Things I Can Do To Make Tomorrow Better:
_____
_____
_____
_____

Date: _____ Wake-Up Time For Today: _____

Hours Slept Last Night: _____

My Mood:

Morning

Afternoon

Evening

How I Feel Today?
- ❏ Anger/frustration
- ❏ Appetite- increased or decreased
- ❏ Difficulty concentrating/making decisions
- ❏ Energized
- ❏ Happy
- ❏ Hopeful
- ❏ Hopeless
- ❏ Joyful
- ❏ Lack of motivation
- ❏ No energy fatigue/lethargic
- ❏ Sad and/or tearful
- ❏ _____
- ❏ _____
- ❏ _____
- ❏ _____

Exercise
_____
_____
_____
_____

Food & Beverage

Breakfast
_____
_____

Lunch
_____
_____

Supper
_____
_____

Snacks
_____
_____

Water

Positive Things That Happened Today:

_____
_____
_____
_____
_____

Is There Anything I Could Have Done To Improve My Day:

_____
_____
_____
_____
_____

Today, I Am Grateful For:

_____
_____
_____
_____
_____

Positive Affirmations:

_____
_____
_____
_____
_____

Goals/Things I Can Do To Make Tomorrow Better:

_____
_____
_____
_____

Date: _____   Wake-Up Time For Today: _____
Hours Slept Last Night:_____

My Mood:

Morning

Afternoon   **Evening**

How I Feel Today?
- ❏ Anger/frustration
- ❏ Appetite- increased or decreased
- ❏ Difficulty concentrating/making decisions
- ❏ Energized
- ❏ Happy
- ❏ Hopeful
- ❏ Hopeless
- ❏ Joyful
- ❏ Lack of motivation
- ❏ No energy fatigue/lethargic
- ❏ Sad and/or tearful
- ❏ _____
- ❏ _____
- ❏ _____
- ❏ _____

Exercise
_____
_____
_____
_____

Food & Beverage

Breakfast
_____
_____

Lunch
_____
_____

Supper
_____
_____

Snacks
_____
_____

Water

Positive Things That Happened Today:

_____
_____
_____
_____
_____

Is There Anything I Could Have Done To Improve My Day:

_____
_____
_____
_____
_____

Today, I Am Grateful For:

_____
_____
_____
_____
_____

Positive Affirmations:

_____
_____
_____
_____
_____

Goals/Things I Can Do To Make Tomorrow Better:

_____
_____
_____
_____
_____

Date: _____ Wake-Up Time For Today: _____
Hours Slept Last Night: _____

My Mood:

Morning

Afternoon   **Evening**

How I Feel Today?
- ❏ Anger/frustration
- ❏ Appetite- increased or decreased
- ❏ Difficulty concentrating/making decisions
- ❏ Energized
- ❏ Happy
- ❏ Hopeful
- ❏ Hopeless
- ❏ Joyful
- ❏ Lack of motivation
- ❏ No energy fatigue/lethargic
- ❏ Sad and/or tearful
- ❏ _____
- ❏ _____
- ❏ _____
- ❏ _____

Exercise
_____
_____
_____
_____

Food & Beverage

Breakfast
_____
_____

Lunch
_____
_____

Supper
_____
_____

Snacks
_____
_____

Water

Positive Things That Happened Today:

_____
_____
_____
_____

Is There Anything I Could Have Done To Improve My Day:

_____
_____
_____
_____
_____

Today, I Am Grateful For:

_____
_____
_____
_____
_____

Positive Affirmations:

_____
_____
_____
_____
_____

Goals/Things I Can Do To Make Tomorrow Better:

_____
_____
_____
_____

Date: _____ Wake-Up Time For Today: _____
Hours Slept Last Night:_____

My Mood:

Morning

Afternoon   **Evening**

How I Feel Today?
- ❑ Anger/frustration
- ❑ Appetite- increased or decreased
- ❑ Difficulty concentrating/making decisions
- ❑ Energized
- ❑ Happy
- ❑ Hopeful
- ❑ Hopeless
- ❑ Joyful
- ❑ Lack of motivation
- ❑ No energy fatigue/lethargic
- ❑ Sad and/or tearful
- ❑ _____
- ❑ _____
- ❑ _____
- ❑ _____

Exercise
_____
_____
_____
_____

Food & Beverage

Breakfast
_____
_____

Lunch
_____
_____

Supper
_____
_____

Snacks
_____
_____

Water

Positive Things That Happened Today:

_____
_____
_____
_____
_____

Is There Anything I Could Have Done To Improve My Day:

_____
_____
_____
_____
_____

Today, I Am Grateful For:

_____
_____
_____
_____
_____

Positive Affirmations:

_____
_____
_____
_____
_____

Goals/Things I Can Do To Make Tomorrow Better:

_____
_____
_____
_____
_____

Date: _____ Wake-Up Time For Today: _____
Hours Slept Last Night: _____

My Mood:

Morning

Afternoon   **Evening**

How I Feel Today?
- ❏ Anger/frustration
- ❏ Appetite- increased or decreased
- ❏ Difficulty concentrating/making decisions
- ❏ Energized
- ❏ Happy
- ❏ Hopeful
- ❏ Hopeless
- ❏ Joyful
- ❏ Lack of motivation
- ❏ No energy fatigue/lethargic
- ❏ Sad and/or tearful
- ❏ _____
- ❏ _____
- ❏ _____
- ❏ _____

Exercise
_____
_____
_____
_____

Food & Beverage

Breakfast
_____
_____

Lunch
_____
_____

Supper
_____
_____

Snacks
_____
_____

Water

Positive Things That Happened Today:
_____
_____
_____
_____

Is There Anything I Could Have Done To Improve My Day:
_____
_____
_____
_____
_____

Today, I Am Grateful For:
_____
_____
_____
_____
_____

Positive Affirmations:
_____
_____
_____
_____

Goals/Things I Can Do To Make Tomorrow Better:
_____
_____
_____
_____

Date: _____ Wake-Up Time For Today: _____

Hours Slept Last Night:_____

My Mood:

Morning

Afternoon

Evening

How I Feel Today?

- ❏ Anger/frustration
- ❏ Appetite- increased or decreased
- ❏ Difficulty concentrating/making decisions
- ❏ Energized
- ❏ Happy
- ❏ Hopeful
- ❏ Hopeless
- ❏ Joyful
- ❏ Lack of motivation
- ❏ No energy fatigue/lethargic
- ❏ Sad and/or tearful
- ❏ _____
- ❏ _____
- ❏ _____
- ❏ _____

Exercise

_____
_____
_____
_____

Food & Beverage

Breakfast

_____
_____

Lunch

_____
_____

Supper

_____
_____

Snacks

_____
_____

Water

Positive Things That Happened Today:

_____
_____
_____
_____
_____

Is There Anything I Could Have Done To Improve My Day:

_____
_____
_____
_____
_____

Today, I Am Grateful For:

_____
_____
_____
_____
_____

Positive Affirmations:

_____
_____
_____
_____
_____

Goals/Things I Can Do To Make Tomorrow Better:

_____
_____
_____
_____
_____

Date: _____ Wake-Up Time For Today: _____
Hours Slept Last Night: _____

My Mood:

Morning

Afternoon   **Evening**

How I Feel Today?
- ❏ Anger/frustration
- ❏ Appetite- increased or decreased
- ❏ Difficulty concentrating/making decisions
- ❏ Energized
- ❏ Happy
- ❏ Hopeful
- ❏ Hopeless
- ❏ Joyful
- ❏ Lack of motivation
- ❏ No energy fatigue/lethargic
- ❏ Sad and/or tearful
- ❏ _____
- ❏ _____
- ❏ _____
- ❏ _____

Exercise
_____
_____
_____
_____

Food & Beverage

Breakfast
_____
_____

Lunch
_____
_____

Supper
_____
_____

Snacks
_____
_____

Water

Positive Things That Happened Today:

_____
_____
_____
_____
_____

Is There Anything I Could Have Done To Improve My Day:

_____
_____
_____
_____
_____
_____

Today, I Am Grateful For:

_____
_____
_____
_____
_____

Positive Affirmations:

_____
_____
_____
_____
_____

Goals/Things I Can Do To Make Tomorrow Better:

_____
_____
_____
_____
_____

Date: _____ Wake-Up Time For Today: _____
Hours Slept Last Night:_____

My Mood:

Morning

Afternoon   **Evening**

How I Feel Today?
- ❏ Anger/frustration
- ❏ Appetite- increased or decreased
- ❏ Difficulty concentrating/making decisions
- ❏ Energized
- ❏ Happy
- ❏ Hopeful
- ❏ Hopeless
- ❏ Joyful
- ❏ Lack of motivation
- ❏ No energy fatigue/lethargic
- ❏ Sad and/or tearful
- ❏ _____
- ❏ _____
- ❏ _____
- ❏ _____

Exercise
_____
_____
_____
_____

Food & Beverage

Breakfast
_____
_____

Lunch
_____
_____

Supper
_____
_____

Snacks
_____
_____

Water

Positive Things That Happened Today:

_____
_____
_____
_____
_____

Is There Anything I Could Have Done To Improve My Day:

_____
_____
_____
_____
_____

Today, I Am Grateful For:

_____
_____
_____
_____

Positive Affirmations:

_____
_____
_____
_____

Goals/Things I Can Do To Make Tomorrow Better:

_____
_____
_____
_____

Date: _____ Wake-Up Time For Today: _____
Hours Slept Last Night: _____

My Mood:

Morning

Afternoon

Evening

How I Feel Today?
- ❏ Anger/frustration
- ❏ Appetite- increased or decreased
- ❏ Difficulty concentrating/making decisions
- ❏ Energized
- ❏ Happy
- ❏ Hopeful
- ❏ Hopeless
- ❏ Joyful
- ❏ Lack of motivation
- ❏ No energy fatigue/lethargic
- ❏ Sad and/or tearful
- ❏ _____
- ❏ _____
- ❏ _____
- ❏ _____

Exercise
_____
_____
_____
_____

Food & Beverage

Breakfast
_____
_____

Lunch
_____
_____

Supper
_____
_____

Snacks
_____
_____

Water

Positive Things That Happened Today:
_____
_____
_____
_____

Is There Anything I Could Have Done To Improve My Day:
_____
_____
_____
_____
_____

Today, I Am Grateful For:
_____
_____
_____
_____

Positive Affirmations:
_____
_____
_____
_____

Goals/Things I Can Do To Make Tomorrow Better:
_____
_____
_____
_____

Date: _____ Wake-Up Time For Today: _____

Hours Slept Last Night:_____

My Mood:

Morning

Afternoon

Evening

How I Feel Today?
- ❏ Anger/frustration
- ❏ Appetite- increased or decreased
- ❏ Difficulty concentrating/making decisions
- ❏ Energized
- ❏ Happy
- ❏ Hopeful
- ❏ Hopeless
- ❏ Joyful
- ❏ Lack of motivation
- ❏ No energy fatigue/lethargic
- ❏ Sad and/or tearful
- ❏ _____
- ❏ _____
- ❏ _____
- ❏ _____

Exercise
_____
_____
_____
_____

Food & Beverage

Breakfast
_____
_____

Lunch
_____
_____

Supper
_____
_____

Snacks
_____
_____

Water

Positive Things That Happened Today:

_____
_____
_____
_____
_____

Is There Anything I Could Have Done To Improve My Day:

_____
_____
_____
_____
_____

Today, I Am Grateful For:

_____
_____
_____
_____
_____

Positive Affirmations:

_____
_____
_____
_____
_____

Goals/Things I Can Do To Make Tomorrow Better:

_____
_____
_____
_____
_____

Date: _____ Wake-Up Time For Today: _____

Hours Slept Last Night:_____

My Mood:

Morning

Afternoon   **Evening**

How I Feel Today?

- ❏ Anger/frustration
- ❏ Appetite- increased or decreased
- ❏ Difficulty concentrating/making decisions
- ❏ Energized
- ❏ Happy
- ❏ Hopeful
- ❏ Hopeless
- ❏ Joyful
- ❏ Lack of motivation
- ❏ No energy fatigue/lethargic
- ❏ Sad and/or tearful
- ❏ _____
- ❏ _____
- ❏ _____
- ❏ _____

Exercise
_____
_____
_____
_____

Food & Beverage

Breakfast
_____
_____

Lunch
_____
_____

Supper
_____
_____

Snacks
_____
_____

Water

Positive Things That Happened Today:

_____
_____
_____
_____

Is There Anything I Could Have Done To Improve My Day:

_____
_____
_____
_____
_____

Today, I Am Grateful For:

_____
_____
_____
_____
_____

Positive Affirmations:

_____
_____
_____
_____
_____

Goals/Things I Can Do To Make Tomorrow Better:

_____
_____
_____
_____

Date: _____ Wake-Up Time For Today: _____
Hours Slept Last Night:_____

My Mood:

Morning

Afternoon   **Evening**

How I Feel Today?
- ❏ Anger/frustration
- ❏ Appetite- increased or decreased
- ❏ Difficulty concentrating/making decisions
- ❏ Energized
- ❏ Happy
- ❏ Hopeful
- ❏ Hopeless
- ❏ Joyful
- ❏ Lack of motivation
- ❏ No energy fatigue/lethargic
- ❏ Sad and/or tearful
- ❏ _____
- ❏ _____
- ❏ _____
- ❏ _____

Exercise
_____
_____
_____
_____

Food & Beverage

Breakfast
_____
_____

Lunch
_____
_____

Supper
_____
_____

Snacks
_____
_____

Water

Positive Things That Happened Today:

_____
_____
_____
_____
_____

Is There Anything I Could Have Done To Improve My Day:

_____
_____
_____
_____
_____

Today, I Am Grateful For:

_____
_____
_____
_____

Positive Affirmations:

_____
_____
_____
_____

Goals/Things I Can Do To Make Tomorrow Better:

_____
_____
_____
_____

Date: _____ Wake-Up Time For Today: _____

Hours Slept Last Night: _____

My Mood:

Morning

Afternoon

Evening

How I Feel Today?

- ❏ Anger/frustration
- ❏ Appetite- increased or decreased
- ❏ Difficulty concentrating/making decisions
- ❏ Energized
- ❏ Happy
- ❏ Hopeful
- ❏ Hopeless
- ❏ Joyful
- ❏ Lack of motivation
- ❏ No energy fatigue/lethargic
- ❏ Sad and/or tearful
- ❏ _____
- ❏ _____
- ❏ _____
- ❏ _____

Exercise

_____
_____
_____
_____

Food & Beverage

Breakfast
_____
_____

Lunch
_____
_____

Supper
_____
_____

Snacks
_____
_____

Water

Positive Things That Happened Today:

_____
_____
_____
_____
_____

Is There Anything I Could Have Done To Improve My Day:

_____
_____
_____
_____
_____
_____

Today, I Am Grateful For:

_____
_____
_____
_____
_____
_____

Positive Affirmations:

_____
_____
_____
_____
_____
_____

Goals/Things I Can Do To Make Tomorrow Better:

_____
_____
_____
_____

Date: _____ Wake-Up Time For Today: _____
Hours Slept Last Night:_____

My Mood:

Morning

Afternoon

Evening

How I Feel Today?
- ❏ Anger/frustration
- ❏ Appetite- increased or decreased
- ❏ Difficulty concentrating/making decisions
- ❏ Energized
- ❏ Happy
- ❏ Hopeful
- ❏ Hopeless
- ❏ Joyful
- ❏ Lack of motivation
- ❏ No energy fatigue/lethargic
- ❏ Sad and/or tearful
- ❏ _____
- ❏ _____
- ❏ _____
- ❏ _____

Exercise
_____
_____
_____
_____

Food & Beverage

Breakfast
_____
_____

Lunch
_____
_____

Supper
_____
_____

Snacks
_____
_____

Water

Positive Things That Happened Today:

_____
_____
_____
_____
_____

Is There Anything I Could Have Done To Improve My Day:

_____
_____
_____
_____
_____

Today, I Am Grateful For:

_____
_____
_____
_____
_____

Positive Affirmations:

_____
_____
_____
_____
_____

Goals/Things I Can Do To Make Tomorrow Better:

_____
_____
_____
_____

Date: _____ Wake-Up Time For Today: _____
Hours Slept Last Night:_____

My Mood:

Morning

Afternoon

Evening

How I Feel Today?
- ❏ Anger/frustration
- ❏ Appetite- increased or decreased
- ❏ Difficulty concentrating/making decisions
- ❏ Energized
- ❏ Happy
- ❏ Hopeful
- ❏ Hopeless
- ❏ Joyful
- ❏ Lack of motivation
- ❏ No energy fatigue/lethargic
- ❏ Sad and/or tearful
- ❏ _____
- ❏ _____
- ❏ _____
- ❏ _____

Exercise
_____
_____
_____
_____

Food & Beverage

Breakfast
_____
_____

Lunch
_____
_____

Supper
_____
_____

Snacks
_____
_____

Water

Positive Things That Happened Today:
_____
_____
_____
_____
_____

Is There Anything I Could Have Done To Improve My Day:
_____
_____
_____
_____
_____

Today, I Am Grateful For:
_____
_____
_____
_____
_____

Positive Affirmations:
_____
_____
_____
_____
_____

Goals/Things I Can Do To Make Tomorrow Better:
_____
_____
_____
_____

Date: _____ Wake-Up Time For Today: _____
Hours Slept Last Night:_____

My Mood:

Morning

Afternoon

Evening

How I Feel Today?
- ❏ Anger/frustration
- ❏ Appetite- increased or decreased
- ❏ Difficulty concentrating/making decisions
- ❏ Energized
- ❏ Happy
- ❏ Hopeful
- ❏ Hopeless
- ❏ Joyful
- ❏ Lack of motivation
- ❏ No energy fatigue/lethargic
- ❏ Sad and/or tearful
- ❏ _____
- ❏ _____
- ❏ _____
- ❏ _____

Exercise
_____
_____
_____
_____

Food & Beverage

Breakfast
_____
_____

Lunch
_____
_____

Supper
_____
_____

Snacks
_____
_____

Water

Positive Things That Happened Today:

_____
_____
_____
_____
_____

Is There Anything I Could Have Done To Improve My Day:

_____
_____
_____
_____
_____

Today, I Am Grateful For:

_____
_____
_____
_____
_____

Positive Affirmations:

_____
_____
_____
_____
_____

Goals/Things I Can Do To Make Tomorrow Better:

_____
_____
_____
_____
_____

Date: _____ Wake-Up Time For Today: _____
Hours Slept Last Night: _____

My Mood:

Morning

Afternoon   **Evening**

How I Feel Today?
- ❑ Anger/frustration
- ❑ Appetite- increased or decreased
- ❑ Difficulty concentrating/making decisions
- ❑ Energized
- ❑ Happy
- ❑ Hopeful
- ❑ Hopeless
- ❑ Joyful
- ❑ Lack of motivation
- ❑ No energy fatigue/lethargic
- ❑ Sad and/or tearful
- ❑ _____
- ❑ _____
- ❑ _____
- ❑ _____

Exercise
_____
_____
_____
_____

Food & Beverage

Breakfast
_____
_____

Lunch
_____
_____

Supper
_____
_____

Snacks
_____
_____

Water

Positive Things That Happened Today:

_____
_____
_____
_____

Is There Anything I Could Have Done To Improve My Day:

_____
_____
_____
_____
_____

Today, I Am Grateful For:

_____
_____
_____
_____

Positive Affirmations:

_____
_____
_____
_____
_____

Goals/Things I Can Do To Make Tomorrow Better:

_____
_____
_____
_____

Date: _____ Wake-Up Time For Today: _____

Hours Slept Last Night: _____

My Mood:

Morning

Afternoon

Evening

How I Feel Today?
- ❏ Anger/frustration
- ❏ Appetite- increased or decreased
- ❏ Difficulty concentrating/making decisions
- ❏ Energized
- ❏ Happy
- ❏ Hopeful
- ❏ Hopeless
- ❏ Joyful
- ❏ Lack of motivation
- ❏ No energy fatigue/lethargic
- ❏ Sad and/or tearful
- ❏ _____
- ❏ _____
- ❏ _____
- ❏ _____

Exercise

_____
_____
_____
_____

Food & Beverage

Breakfast

_____
_____

Lunch

_____
_____

Supper

_____
_____

Snacks

_____
_____

Water

Positive Things That Happened Today:

_____
_____
_____
_____
_____

Is There Anything I Could Have Done To Improve My Day:

_____
_____
_____
_____
_____

Today, I Am Grateful For:

_____
_____
_____
_____
_____

Positive Affirmations:

_____
_____
_____
_____
_____

Goals/Things I Can Do To Make Tomorrow Better:

_____
_____
_____
_____
_____

Date: _____ Wake-Up Time For Today: _____
Hours Slept Last Night:_____

My Mood:

Morning

Afternoon

Evening

How I Feel Today?
- ❏ Anger/frustration
- ❏ Appetite- increased or decreased
- ❏ Difficulty concentrating/making decisions
- ❏ Energized
- ❏ Happy
- ❏ Hopeful
- ❏ Hopeless
- ❏ Joyful
- ❏ Lack of motivation
- ❏ No energy fatigue/lethargic
- ❏ Sad and/or tearful
- ❏ _____
- ❏ _____
- ❏ _____
- ❏ _____

Exercise
_____
_____
_____
_____

Food & Beverage

Breakfast
_____
_____

Lunch
_____
_____

Supper
_____
_____

Snacks
_____
_____

Water

Positive Things That Happened Today:

_____
_____
_____
_____
_____

Is There Anything I Could Have Done To Improve My Day:

_____
_____
_____
_____
_____

Today, I Am Grateful For:

_____
_____
_____
_____
_____

Positive Affirmations:

_____
_____
_____
_____
_____

Goals/Things I Can Do To Make Tomorrow Better:

_____
_____
_____
_____

Date: _____ Wake-Up Time For Today: _____

Hours Slept Last Night:_____

My Mood:

Morning

Afternoon **Evening**

How I Feel Today?
- ❏ Anger/frustration
- ❏ Appetite- increased or decreased
- ❏ Difficulty concentrating/making decisions
- ❏ Energized
- ❏ Happy
- ❏ Hopeful
- ❏ Hopeless
- ❏ Joyful
- ❏ Lack of motivation
- ❏ No energy fatigue/lethargic
- ❏ Sad and/or tearful
- ❏ _____
- ❏ _____
- ❏ _____
- ❏ _____

Exercise
_____
_____
_____
_____

Food & Beverage

Breakfast
_____
_____

Lunch
_____
_____

Supper
_____
_____

Snacks
_____
_____

Water

Positive Things That Happened Today:

_____
_____
_____
_____
_____

Is There Anything I Could Have Done To Improve My Day:

_____
_____
_____
_____
_____

Today, I Am Grateful For:

_____
_____
_____
_____
_____

Positive Affirmations:

_____
_____
_____
_____
_____

Goals/Things I Can Do To Make Tomorrow Better:

_____
_____
_____
_____

Date: _____ Wake-Up Time For Today: _____

Hours Slept Last Night: _____

My Mood:

Morning

Afternoon   **Evening**

How I Feel Today?
- ❏ Anger/frustration
- ❏ Appetite- increased or decreased
- ❏ Difficulty concentrating/making decisions
- ❏ Energized
- ❏ Happy
- ❏ Hopeful
- ❏ Hopeless
- ❏ Joyful
- ❏ Lack of motivation
- ❏ No energy fatigue/lethargic
- ❏ Sad and/or tearful
- ❏ _____
- ❏ _____
- ❏ _____
- ❏ _____

Exercise
_____
_____
_____
_____

Food & Beverage

Breakfast
_____
_____

Lunch
_____
_____

Supper
_____
_____

Snacks
_____
_____

Water

Positive Things That Happened Today:

_____
_____
_____
_____
_____

Is There Anything I Could Have Done To Improve My Day:

_____
_____
_____
_____
_____
_____

Today, I Am Grateful For:

_____
_____
_____
_____
_____
_____

Positive Affirmations:

_____
_____
_____
_____
_____

Goals/Things I Can Do To Make Tomorrow Better:

_____
_____
_____
_____
_____

Date: _____ Wake-Up Time For Today: _____

Hours Slept Last Night:_____

My Mood:

Morning

Afternoon   **Evening**

How I Feel Today?
- ❏ Anger/frustration
- ❏ Appetite- increased or decreased
- ❏ Difficulty concentrating/making decisions
- ❏ Energized
- ❏ Happy
- ❏ Hopeful
- ❏ Hopeless
- ❏ Joyful
- ❏ Lack of motivation
- ❏ No energy fatigue/lethargic
- ❏ Sad and/or tearful
- ❏ _____
- ❏ _____
- ❏ _____
- ❏ _____

Exercise
_____
_____
_____
_____

Food & Beverage

Breakfast
_____
_____

Lunch
_____
_____

Supper
_____
_____

Snacks
_____
_____

Water

Positive Things That Happened Today:

_____
_____
_____
_____
_____

Is There Anything I Could Have Done To Improve My Day:

_____
_____
_____
_____
_____

Today, I Am Grateful For:

_____
_____
_____
_____
_____

Positive Affirmations:

_____
_____
_____
_____
_____

Goals/Things I Can Do To Make Tomorrow Better:

_____
_____
_____
_____
_____

Date: _____ Wake-Up Time For Today: _____

Hours Slept Last Night: _____

My Mood:

Morning

Afternoon

Evening

How I Feel Today?
- ❏ Anger/frustration
- ❏ Appetite- increased or decreased
- ❏ Difficulty concentrating/making decisions
- ❏ Energized
- ❏ Happy
- ❏ Hopeful
- ❏ Hopeless
- ❏ Joyful
- ❏ Lack of motivation
- ❏ No energy fatigue/lethargic
- ❏ Sad and/or tearful
- ❏ _____
- ❏ _____
- ❏ _____
- ❏ _____

Exercise

_____
_____
_____
_____

Food & Beverage

Breakfast

_____
_____

Lunch

_____
_____

Supper

_____
_____

Snacks

_____
_____

Water

Positive Things That Happened Today:

_____
_____
_____
_____
_____

Is There Anything I Could Have Done To Improve My Day:

_____
_____
_____
_____
_____

Today, I Am Grateful For:

_____
_____
_____
_____

Positive Affirmations:

_____
_____
_____
_____

Goals/Things I Can Do To Make Tomorrow Better:

_____
_____
_____
_____

Date: _____ Wake-Up Time For Today: _____

Hours Slept Last Night:_____

My Mood:

Morning

Afternoon **Evening**

How I Feel Today?
- ❏ Anger/frustration
- ❏ Appetite- increased or decreased
- ❏ Difficulty concentrating/making decisions
- ❏ Energized
- ❏ Happy
- ❏ Hopeful
- ❏ Hopeless
- ❏ Joyful
- ❏ Lack of motivation
- ❏ No energy fatigue/lethargic
- ❏ Sad and/or tearful
- ❏ _____
- ❏ _____
- ❏ _____
- ❏ _____

Exercise
_____
_____
_____
_____

Food & Beverage

Breakfast
_____
_____

Lunch
_____
_____

Supper
_____
_____

Snacks
_____
_____

Water

Positive Things That Happened Today:

_____
_____
_____
_____

Is There Anything I Could Have Done To Improve My Day:

_____
_____
_____
_____

Today, I Am Grateful For:

_____
_____
_____
_____

Positive Affirmations:

_____
_____
_____
_____

Goals/Things I Can Do To Make Tomorrow Better:

_____
_____
_____
_____

Date: _____ Wake-Up Time For Today: _____
Hours Slept Last Night:_____

My Mood:

Morning

Afternoon **Evening**

How I Feel Today?
- ❏ Anger/frustration
- ❏ Appetite- increased or decreased
- ❏ Difficulty concentrating/making decisions
- ❏ Energized
- ❏ Happy
- ❏ Hopeful
- ❏ Hopeless
- ❏ Joyful
- ❏ Lack of motivation
- ❏ No energy fatigue/lethargic
- ❏ Sad and/or tearful
- ❏ _____
- ❏ _____
- ❏ _____
- ❏ _____

Exercise
_____
_____
_____
_____

Food & Beverage

Breakfast
_____
_____

Lunch
_____
_____

Supper
_____
_____

Snacks
_____
_____

Water

Positive Things That Happened Today:

_____
_____
_____
_____
_____

Is There Anything I Could Have Done To Improve My Day:

_____
_____
_____
_____
_____

Today, I Am Grateful For:

_____
_____
_____
_____
_____

Positive Affirmations:

_____
_____
_____
_____
_____

Goals/Things I Can Do To Make Tomorrow Better:

_____
_____
_____
_____
_____

Date: _____ Wake-Up Time For Today: _____
Hours Slept Last Night: _____

My Mood:

Morning

Afternoon

Evening

How I Feel Today?
- ❑ Anger/frustration
- ❑ Appetite- increased or decreased
- ❑ Difficulty concentrating/making decisions
- ❑ Energized
- ❑ Happy
- ❑ Hopeful
- ❑ Hopeless
- ❑ Joyful
- ❑ Lack of motivation
- ❑ No energy fatigue/lethargic
- ❑ Sad and/or tearful
- ❑ _____
- ❑ _____
- ❑ _____
- ❑ _____

Exercise
_____
_____
_____
_____

Food & Beverage

Breakfast
_____
_____

Lunch
_____
_____

Supper
_____
_____

Snacks
_____
_____

Water

Positive Things That Happened Today:

_____
_____
_____
_____
_____

Is There Anything I Could Have Done To Improve My Day:

_____
_____
_____
_____
_____

Today, I Am Grateful For:

_____
_____
_____
_____
_____

Positive Affirmations:

_____
_____
_____
_____
_____

Goals/Things I Can Do To Make Tomorrow Better:

_____
_____
_____
_____

Date: _____ Wake-Up Time For Today: _____
Hours Slept Last Night:_____

My Mood:

Morning

Afternoon   **Evening**

How I Feel Today?
- ❏ Anger/frustration
- ❏ Appetite- increased or decreased
- ❏ Difficulty concentrating/making decisions
- ❏ Energized
- ❏ Happy
- ❏ Hopeful
- ❏ Hopeless
- ❏ Joyful
- ❏ Lack of motivation
- ❏ No energy fatigue/lethargic
- ❏ Sad and/or tearful
- ❏ _____
- ❏ _____
- ❏ _____
- ❏ _____

Exercise
_____
_____
_____
_____

Food & Beverage

Breakfast
_____
_____

Lunch
_____
_____

Supper
_____
_____

Snacks
_____
_____

Water

Positive Things That Happened Today:

_____
_____
_____
_____
_____

Is There Anything I Could Have Done To Improve My Day:

_____
_____
_____
_____
_____

Today, I Am Grateful For:

_____
_____
_____
_____
_____

Positive Affirmations:

_____
_____
_____
_____
_____

Goals/Things I Can Do To Make Tomorrow Better:

_____
_____
_____
_____

Date: _____ Wake-Up Time For Today: _____
Hours Slept Last Night: _____

My Mood:

Morning

Afternoon

Evening

How I Feel Today?
- ❏ Anger/frustration
- ❏ Appetite- increased or decreased
- ❏ Difficulty concentrating/making decisions
- ❏ Energized
- ❏ Happy
- ❏ Hopeful
- ❏ Hopeless
- ❏ Joyful
- ❏ Lack of motivation
- ❏ No energy fatigue/lethargic
- ❏ Sad and/or tearful
- ❏ _____
- ❏ _____
- ❏ _____
- ❏ _____

Exercise
_____
_____
_____
_____

Food & Beverage

Breakfast
_____
_____

Lunch
_____
_____

Supper
_____
_____

Snacks
_____
_____

Water

Positive Things That Happened Today:

_____
_____
_____
_____
_____

Is There Anything I Could Have Done To Improve My Day:

_____
_____
_____
_____
_____

Today, I Am Grateful For:

_____
_____
_____
_____
_____

Positive Affirmations:

_____
_____
_____
_____
_____

Goals/Things I Can Do To Make Tomorrow Better:

_____
_____
_____
_____
_____

Date: _____ Wake-Up Time For Today: _____

Hours Slept Last Night:_____

My Mood:

Morning

Afternoon　　　　　　　　　　　　　　**Evening**

How I Feel Today?

- ❏ Anger/frustration
- ❏ Appetite- increased or decreased
- ❏ Difficulty concentrating/making decisions
- ❏ Energized
- ❏ Happy
- ❏ Hopeful
- ❏ Hopeless
- ❏ Joyful
- ❏ Lack of motivation
- ❏ No energy fatigue/lethargic
- ❏ Sad and/or tearful
- ❏ _____
- ❏ _____
- ❏ _____
- ❏ _____

Exercise
_____
_____
_____
_____

Food & Beverage

Breakfast
_____
_____

Lunch
_____
_____

Supper
_____
_____

Snacks
_____
_____

Water

Positive Things That Happened Today:

_____
_____
_____
_____
_____

Is There Anything I Could Have Done To Improve My Day:

_____
_____
_____
_____
_____

Today, I Am Grateful For:

_____
_____
_____
_____
_____

Positive Affirmations:

_____
_____
_____
_____

Goals/Things I Can Do To Make Tomorrow Better:

_____
_____
_____
_____

Date: _____   Wake-Up Time For Today: _____
Hours Slept Last Night:_____

My Mood:

Morning

Afternoon   **Evening**

How I Feel Today?
- ❑ Anger/frustration
- ❑ Appetite- increased or decreased
- ❑ Difficulty concentrating/making decisions
- ❑ Energized
- ❑ Happy
- ❑ Hopeful
- ❑ Hopeless
- ❑ Joyful
- ❑ Lack of motivation
- ❑ No energy fatigue/lethargic
- ❑ Sad and/or tearful
- ❑ _____
- ❑ _____
- ❑ _____
- ❑ _____

Exercise
_____
_____
_____
_____

Food & Beverage

Breakfast
_____
_____

Lunch
_____
_____

Supper
_____
_____

Snacks
_____
_____

Water

Positive Things That Happened Today:

_____
_____
_____
_____
_____

Is There Anything I Could Have Done To Improve My Day:

_____
_____
_____
_____
_____

Today, I Am Grateful For:

_____
_____
_____
_____
_____

Positive Affirmations:

_____
_____
_____
_____
_____

Goals/Things I Can Do To Make Tomorrow Better:

_____
_____
_____
_____
_____

Date: _____ Wake-Up Time For Today: _____
Hours Slept Last Night: _____

My Mood:

Morning

Afternoon

Evening

How I Feel Today?
- ❏ Anger/frustration
- ❏ Appetite- increased or decreased
- ❏ Difficulty concentrating/making decisions
- ❏ Energized
- ❏ Happy
- ❏ Hopeful
- ❏ Hopeless
- ❏ Joyful
- ❏ Lack of motivation
- ❏ No energy fatigue/lethargic
- ❏ Sad and/or tearful
- ❏ _____
- ❏ _____
- ❏ _____
- ❏ _____

Exercise
_____
_____
_____
_____

Food & Beverage

Breakfast
_____
_____

Lunch
_____
_____

Supper
_____
_____

Snacks
_____
_____

Water

Positive Things That Happened Today:

_____
_____
_____
_____

Is There Anything I Could Have Done To Improve My Day:

_____
_____
_____
_____
_____

Today, I Am Grateful For:

_____
_____
_____
_____
_____

Positive Affirmations:

_____
_____
_____
_____
_____

Goals/Things I Can Do To Make Tomorrow Better:

_____
_____
_____
_____

Date: _____ Wake-Up Time For Today: _____
Hours Slept Last Night:_____

My Mood:

Morning

Afternoon

Evening

How I Feel Today?
- ❑ Anger/frustration
- ❑ Appetite- increased or decreased
- ❑ Difficulty concentrating/making decisions
- ❑ Energized
- ❑ Happy
- ❑ Hopeful
- ❑ Hopeless
- ❑ Joyful
- ❑ Lack of motivation
- ❑ No energy fatigue/lethargic
- ❑ Sad and/or tearful
- ❑ _____
- ❑ _____
- ❑ _____
- ❑ _____

Exercise
_____
_____
_____
_____

Food & Beverage

Breakfast
_____
_____

Lunch
_____
_____

Supper
_____
_____

Snacks
_____
_____

Water

Positive Things That Happened Today:

_____
_____
_____
_____
_____

Is There Anything I Could Have Done To Improve My Day:

_____
_____
_____
_____
_____

Today, I Am Grateful For:

_____
_____
_____
_____
_____

Positive Affirmations:

_____
_____
_____
_____
_____

Goals/Things I Can Do To Make Tomorrow Better:

_____
_____
_____
_____
_____

Date: _____ Wake-Up Time For Today: _____
Hours Slept Last Night: _____

My Mood:

Morning

Afternoon   **Evening**

How I Feel Today?
- ❑ Anger/frustration
- ❑ Appetite- increased or decreased
- ❑ Difficulty concentrating/making decisions
- ❑ Energized
- ❑ Happy
- ❑ Hopeful
- ❑ Hopeless
- ❑ Joyful
- ❑ Lack of motivation
- ❑ No energy fatigue/lethargic
- ❑ Sad and/or tearful
- ❑ _____
- ❑ _____
- ❑ _____
- ❑ _____

Exercise
_____
_____
_____
_____

Food & Beverage

Breakfast
_____
_____

Lunch
_____
_____

Supper
_____
_____

Snacks
_____
_____

Water

Positive Things That Happened Today:

_____
_____
_____
_____

Is There Anything I Could Have Done To Improve My Day:

_____
_____
_____
_____
_____

Today, I Am Grateful For:

_____
_____
_____
_____
_____

Positive Affirmations:

_____
_____
_____
_____
_____

Goals/Things I Can Do To Make Tomorrow Better:

_____
_____
_____
_____

Date: _____ Wake-Up Time For Today: _____
Hours Slept Last Night: _____

My Mood:

Morning

Afternoon

Evening

How I Feel Today?
- ❏ Anger/frustration
- ❏ Appetite- increased or decreased
- ❏ Difficulty concentrating/making decisions
- ❏ Energized
- ❏ Happy
- ❏ Hopeful
- ❏ Hopeless
- ❏ Joyful
- ❏ Lack of motivation
- ❏ No energy fatigue/lethargic
- ❏ Sad and/or tearful
- ❏ _____
- ❏ _____
- ❏ _____
- ❏ _____

Exercise
_____
_____
_____
_____

Food & Beverage

Breakfast
_____
_____

Lunch
_____
_____

Supper
_____
_____

Snacks
_____
_____

Water

Positive Things That Happened Today:

_____
_____
_____
_____
_____

Is There Anything I Could Have Done To Improve My Day:

_____
_____
_____
_____
_____

Today, I Am Grateful For:

_____
_____
_____
_____
_____

Positive Affirmations:

_____
_____
_____
_____
_____

Goals/Things I Can Do To Make Tomorrow Better:

_____
_____
_____
_____
_____

Date: _____ Wake-Up Time For Today: _____
Hours Slept Last Night: _____

My Mood:

Morning

Afternoon

Evening

How I Feel Today?
- ☐ Anger/frustration
- ☐ Appetite- increased or decreased
- ☐ Difficulty concentrating/making decisions
- ☐ Energized
- ☐ Happy
- ☐ Hopeful
- ☐ Hopeless
- ☐ Joyful
- ☐ Lack of motivation
- ☐ No energy fatigue/lethargic
- ☐ Sad and/or tearful
- ☐ _____
- ☐ _____
- ☐ _____
- ☐ _____

Exercise
_____
_____
_____
_____

Food & Beverage

Breakfast
_____
_____

Lunch
_____
_____

Supper
_____
_____

Snacks
_____
_____

Water

Positive Things That Happened Today:

_____
_____
_____
_____
_____

Is There Anything I Could Have Done To Improve My Day:

_____
_____
_____
_____
_____

Today, I Am Grateful For:

_____
_____
_____
_____
_____

Positive Affirmations:

_____
_____
_____
_____
_____

Goals/Things I Can Do To Make Tomorrow Better:

_____
_____
_____
_____
_____

Date: _____ Wake-Up Time For Today: _____
Hours Slept Last Night:_____

My Mood:

Morning

Afternoon   **Evening**

How I Feel Today?
- ❏ Anger/frustration
- ❏ Appetite- increased or decreased
- ❏ Difficulty concentrating/making decisions
- ❏ Energized
- ❏ Happy
- ❏ Hopeful
- ❏ Hopeless
- ❏ Joyful
- ❏ Lack of motivation
- ❏ No energy fatigue/lethargic
- ❏ Sad and/or tearful
- ❏ _____
- ❏ _____
- ❏ _____
- ❏ _____

Exercise
_____
_____
_____
_____

Food & Beverage

Breakfast
_____
_____

Lunch
_____
_____

Supper
_____
_____

Snacks
_____
_____

Water

Positive Things That Happened Today:

_____
_____
_____
_____
_____

Is There Anything I Could Have Done To Improve My Day:

_____
_____
_____
_____
_____

Today, I Am Grateful For:

_____
_____
_____
_____
_____

Positive Affirmations:

_____
_____
_____
_____
_____

Goals/Things I Can Do To Make Tomorrow Better:

_____
_____
_____
_____
_____

Date: _____ Wake-Up Time For Today: _____
Hours Slept Last Night: _____

My Mood:

Morning

Afternoon

Evening

How I Feel Today?

- ❑ Anger/frustration
- ❑ Appetite- increased or decreased
- ❑ Difficulty concentrating/making decisions
- ❑ Energized
- ❑ Happy
- ❑ Hopeful
- ❑ Hopeless
- ❑ Joyful
- ❑ Lack of motivation
- ❑ No energy fatigue/lethargic
- ❑ Sad and/or tearful
- ❑ _____
- ❑ _____
- ❑ _____
- ❑ _____

Exercise

_____
_____
_____
_____

Food & Beverage

Breakfast

_____
_____

Lunch

_____
_____

Supper

_____
_____

Snacks

_____
_____

Water

Positive Things That Happened Today:

_____
_____
_____
_____
_____

Is There Anything I Could Have Done To Improve My Day:

_____
_____
_____
_____
_____
_____

Today, I Am Grateful For:

_____
_____
_____
_____
_____
_____

Positive Affirmations:

_____
_____
_____
_____
_____
_____

Goals/Things I Can Do To Make Tomorrow Better:

_____
_____
_____
_____
_____

Date: _____ Wake-Up Time For Today: _____
Hours Slept Last Night:_____

My Mood:

Morning

Afternoon **Evening**

How I Feel Today?
- ❏ Anger/frustration
- ❏ Appetite- increased or decreased
- ❏ Difficulty concentrating/making decisions
- ❏ Energized
- ❏ Happy
- ❏ Hopeful
- ❏ Hopeless
- ❏ Joyful
- ❏ Lack of motivation
- ❏ No energy fatigue/lethargic
- ❏ Sad and/or tearful
- ❏ _____
- ❏ _____
- ❏ _____
- ❏ _____

Exercise
_____
_____
_____
_____

Food & Beverage

Breakfast
_____
_____

Lunch
_____
_____

Supper
_____
_____

Snacks
_____
_____

Water

Positive Things That Happened Today:

_____
_____
_____
_____

Is There Anything I Could Have Done To Improve My Day:

_____
_____
_____
_____

Today, I Am Grateful For:

_____
_____
_____
_____

Positive Affirmations:

_____
_____
_____
_____

Goals/Things I Can Do To Make Tomorrow Better:

_____
_____
_____
_____

Date: _____ Wake-Up Time For Today: _____
Hours Slept Last Night: _____

My Mood:

Morning

Afternoon

Evening

How I Feel Today?
- ☐ Anger/frustration
- ☐ Appetite- increased or decreased
- ☐ Difficulty concentrating/making decisions
- ☐ Energized
- ☐ Happy
- ☐ Hopeful
- ☐ Hopeless
- ☐ Joyful
- ☐ Lack of motivation
- ☐ No energy fatigue/lethargic
- ☐ Sad and/or tearful
- ☐ _____
- ☐ _____
- ☐ _____
- ☐ _____

Exercise
_____
_____
_____
_____

Food & Beverage

Breakfast
_____
_____

Lunch
_____
_____

Supper
_____
_____

Snacks
_____
_____

Water

Positive Things That Happened Today:

_____
_____
_____
_____
_____

Is There Anything I Could Have Done To Improve My Day:

_____
_____
_____
_____
_____

Today, I Am Grateful For:

_____
_____
_____
_____
_____

Positive Affirmations:

_____
_____
_____
_____
_____

Goals/Things I Can Do To Make Tomorrow Better:

_____
_____
_____
_____
_____

Date: _____ Wake-Up Time For Today: _____
Hours Slept Last Night:_____

My Mood:

Morning

Afternoon

Evening

How I Feel Today?
- ❏ Anger/frustration
- ❏ Appetite- increased or decreased
- ❏ Difficulty concentrating/making decisions
- ❏ Energized
- ❏ Happy
- ❏ Hopeful
- ❏ Hopeless
- ❏ Joyful
- ❏ Lack of motivation
- ❏ No energy fatigue/lethargic
- ❏ Sad and/or tearful
- ❏ _____
- ❏ _____
- ❏ _____
- ❏ _____

Exercise
_____
_____
_____
_____

Food & Beverage

Breakfast
_____
_____

Lunch
_____
_____

Supper
_____
_____

Snacks
_____
_____

Water

Positive Things That Happened Today:

_____
_____
_____
_____
_____

Is There Anything I Could Have Done To Improve My Day:

_____
_____
_____
_____
_____

Today, I Am Grateful For:

_____
_____
_____
_____
_____

Positive Affirmations:

_____
_____
_____
_____
_____

Goals/Things I Can Do To Make Tomorrow Better:

_____
_____
_____
_____
_____

Date: _____ Wake-Up Time For Today: _____

Hours Slept Last Night: _____

My Mood:

Morning

Afternoon

Evening

How I Feel Today?
- ❑ Anger/frustration
- ❑ Appetite- increased or decreased
- ❑ Difficulty concentrating/making decisions
- ❑ Energized
- ❑ Happy
- ❑ Hopeful
- ❑ Hopeless
- ❑ Joyful
- ❑ Lack of motivation
- ❑ No energy fatigue/lethargic
- ❑ Sad and/or tearful
- ❑ _____
- ❑ _____
- ❑ _____
- ❑ _____

Exercise
_____
_____
_____
_____

Food & Beverage

Breakfast
_____
_____

Lunch
_____
_____

Supper
_____
_____

Snacks
_____
_____

Water

Positive Things That Happened Today:

_____
_____
_____
_____
_____

Is There Anything I Could Have Done To Improve My Day:

_____
_____
_____
_____
_____

Today, I Am Grateful For:

_____
_____
_____
_____
_____

Positive Affirmations:

_____
_____
_____
_____
_____

Goals/Things I Can Do To Make Tomorrow Better:

_____
_____
_____
_____
_____

Date: _____ Wake-Up Time For Today: _____
Hours Slept Last Night:_____

My Mood:

Morning

Afternoon   **Evening**

How I Feel Today?
- ❏ Anger/frustration
- ❏ Appetite- increased or decreased
- ❏ Difficulty concentrating/making decisions
- ❏ Energized
- ❏ Happy
- ❏ Hopeful
- ❏ Hopeless
- ❏ Joyful
- ❏ Lack of motivation
- ❏ No energy fatigue/lethargic
- ❏ Sad and/or tearful
- ❏ _____
- ❏ _____
- ❏ _____
- ❏ _____

Exercise
_____
_____
_____
_____

Food & Beverage

Breakfast
_____
_____

Lunch
_____
_____

Supper
_____
_____

Snacks
_____
_____

Water

Positive Things That Happened Today:

_____
_____
_____
_____

Is There Anything I Could Have Done To Improve My Day:

_____
_____
_____
_____
_____
_____

Today, I Am Grateful For:

_____
_____
_____
_____
_____

Positive Affirmations:

_____
_____
_____
_____
_____

Goals/Things I Can Do To Make Tomorrow Better:

_____
_____
_____
_____

Date: _____ Wake-Up Time For Today: _____
Hours Slept Last Night:_____

My Mood:

Morning

Afternoon   **Evening**

How I Feel Today?
- ❏ Anger/frustration
- ❏ Appetite- increased or decreased
- ❏ Difficulty concentrating/making decisions
- ❏ Energized
- ❏ Happy
- ❏ Hopeful
- ❏ Hopeless
- ❏ Joyful
- ❏ Lack of motivation
- ❏ No energy fatigue/lethargic
- ❏ Sad and/or tearful
- ❏ _____
- ❏ _____
- ❏ _____
- ❏ _____

Exercise
_____
_____
_____
_____

Food & Beverage

Breakfast
_____
_____

Lunch
_____
_____

Supper
_____
_____

Snacks
_____
_____

Water

Positive Things That Happened Today:

_____
_____
_____
_____

Is There Anything I Could Have Done To Improve My Day:

_____
_____
_____
_____
_____

Today, I Am Grateful For:

_____
_____
_____
_____
_____

Positive Affirmations:

_____
_____
_____
_____
_____

Goals/Things I Can Do To Make Tomorrow Better:

_____
_____
_____
_____

Date: _____ Wake-Up Time For Today: _____
Hours Slept Last Night: _____

My Mood:

Morning

Afternoon

Evening

How I Feel Today?
- ❏ Anger/frustration
- ❏ Appetite- increased or decreased
- ❏ Difficulty concentrating/making decisions
- ❏ Energized
- ❏ Happy
- ❏ Hopeful
- ❏ Hopeless
- ❏ Joyful
- ❏ Lack of motivation
- ❏ No energy fatigue/lethargic
- ❏ Sad and/or tearful
- ❏ _____
- ❏ _____
- ❏ _____
- ❏ _____

Exercise
_____
_____
_____
_____

Food & Beverage

Breakfast
_____
_____

Lunch
_____
_____

Supper
_____
_____

Snacks
_____
_____

Water

Positive Things That Happened Today:

_____
_____
_____
_____
_____

Is There Anything I Could Have Done To Improve My Day:

_____
_____
_____
_____
_____

Today, I Am Grateful For:

_____
_____
_____
_____
_____

Positive Affirmations:

_____
_____
_____
_____
_____

Goals/Things I Can Do To Make Tomorrow Better:

_____
_____
_____
_____
_____

Date: _____ Wake-Up Time For Today: _____

Hours Slept Last Night:_____

My Mood:

Morning

Afternoon   **Evening**

How I Feel Today?
- ❑ Anger/frustration
- ❑ Appetite- increased or decreased
- ❑ Difficulty concentrating/making decisions
- ❑ Energized
- ❑ Happy
- ❑ Hopeful
- ❑ Hopeless
- ❑ Joyful
- ❑ Lack of motivation
- ❑ No energy fatigue/lethargic
- ❑ Sad and/or tearful
- ❑ _____
- ❑ _____
- ❑ _____
- ❑ _____

Exercise
_____
_____
_____
_____

Food & Beverage

Breakfast
_____
_____

Lunch
_____
_____

Supper
_____
_____

Snacks
_____
_____

Water

Positive Things That Happened Today:

_____
_____
_____
_____

Is There Anything I Could Have Done To Improve My Day:

_____
_____
_____
_____
_____

Today, I Am Grateful For:

_____
_____
_____
_____

Positive Affirmations:

_____
_____
_____
_____

Goals/Things I Can Do To Make Tomorrow Better:

_____
_____
_____
_____

Date: _____ Wake-Up Time For Today: _____
Hours Slept Last Night: _____

My Mood:

Morning

Afternoon

Evening

How I Feel Today?
- ❑ Anger/frustration
- ❑ Appetite- increased or decreased
- ❑ Difficulty concentrating/making decisions
- ❑ Energized
- ❑ Happy
- ❑ Hopeful
- ❑ Hopeless
- ❑ Joyful
- ❑ Lack of motivation
- ❑ No energy fatigue/lethargic
- ❑ Sad and/or tearful
- ❑ _____
- ❑ _____
- ❑ _____
- ❑ _____

Exercise
_____
_____
_____
_____

Food & Beverage

Breakfast
_____
_____

Lunch
_____
_____

Supper
_____
_____

Snacks
_____
_____

Water

Positive Things That Happened Today:

_____
_____
_____
_____
_____

Is There Anything I Could Have Done To Improve My Day:

_____
_____
_____
_____
_____

Today, I Am Grateful For:

_____
_____
_____
_____
_____

Positive Affirmations:

_____
_____
_____
_____
_____

Goals/Things I Can Do To Make Tomorrow Better:

_____
_____
_____
_____
_____

Date: _____ Wake-Up Time For Today: _____

Hours Slept Last Night: _____

My Mood:

Morning

Afternoon   **Evening**

How I Feel Today?
- ❏ Anger/frustration
- ❏ Appetite- increased or decreased
- ❏ Difficulty concentrating/making decisions
- ❏ Energized
- ❏ Happy
- ❏ Hopeful
- ❏ Hopeless
- ❏ Joyful
- ❏ Lack of motivation
- ❏ No energy fatigue/lethargic
- ❏ Sad and/or tearful
- ❏ _____
- ❏ _____
- ❏ _____
- ❏ _____

Exercise
_____
_____
_____
_____

Food & Beverage

Breakfast
_____
_____

Lunch
_____
_____

Supper
_____
_____

Snacks
_____
_____

Water

Positive Things That Happened Today:

_____
_____
_____
_____
_____

Is There Anything I Could Have Done To Improve My Day:

_____
_____
_____
_____
_____
_____

Today, I Am Grateful For:

_____
_____
_____
_____
_____

Positive Affirmations:

_____
_____
_____
_____
_____

Goals/Things I Can Do To Make Tomorrow Better:

_____
_____
_____
_____

Date: _____ Wake-Up Time For Today: _____
Hours Slept Last Night:_____

My Mood:

Morning

Afternoon

Evening

How I Feel Today?
- ❏ Anger/frustration
- ❏ Appetite- increased or decreased
- ❏ Difficulty concentrating/making decisions
- ❏ Energized
- ❏ Happy
- ❏ Hopeful
- ❏ Hopeless
- ❏ Joyful
- ❏ Lack of motivation
- ❏ No energy fatigue/lethargic
- ❏ Sad and/or tearful
- ❏ _____
- ❏ _____
- ❏ _____
- ❏ _____

Exercise
_____
_____
_____
_____

Food & Beverage

Breakfast
_____
_____

Lunch
_____
_____

Supper
_____
_____

Snacks
_____
_____

Water

Positive Things That Happened Today:

_____
_____
_____
_____
_____

Is There Anything I Could Have Done To Improve My Day:

_____
_____
_____
_____
_____

Today, I Am Grateful For:

_____
_____
_____
_____
_____

Positive Affirmations:

_____
_____
_____
_____
_____

Goals/Things I Can Do To Make Tomorrow Better:

_____
_____
_____
_____
_____

Date: _____ Wake-Up Time For Today: _____

Hours Slept Last Night:_____

My Mood:

Morning

Afternoon   **Evening**

How I Feel Today?

- ❑ Anger/frustration
- ❑ Appetite- increased or decreased
- ❑ Difficulty concentrating/making decisions
- ❑ Energized
- ❑ Happy
- ❑ Hopeful
- ❑ Hopeless
- ❑ Joyful
- ❑ Lack of motivation
- ❑ No energy fatigue/lethargic
- ❑ Sad and/or tearful
- ❑ _____
- ❑ _____
- ❑ _____
- ❑ _____

Exercise
_____
_____
_____
_____

Food & Beverage

Breakfast
_____
_____

Lunch
_____
_____

Supper
_____
_____

Snacks
_____
_____

Water

Positive Things That Happened Today:

_____
_____
_____
_____

Is There Anything I Could Have Done To Improve My Day:

_____
_____
_____
_____

Today, I Am Grateful For:

_____
_____
_____
_____

Positive Affirmations:

_____
_____
_____
_____

Goals/Things I Can Do To Make Tomorrow Better:

_____
_____
_____
_____

Date: _____ Wake-Up Time For Today: _____
Hours Slept Last Night:_____

My Mood:

Morning

Afternoon

Evening

How I Feel Today?
- ☐ Anger/frustration
- ☐ Appetite- increased or decreased
- ☐ Difficulty concentrating/making decisions
- ☐ Energized
- ☐ Happy
- ☐ Hopeful
- ☐ Hopeless
- ☐ Joyful
- ☐ Lack of motivation
- ☐ No energy fatigue/lethargic
- ☐ Sad and/or tearful
- ☐ _____
- ☐ _____
- ☐ _____
- ☐ _____

Exercise
_____
_____
_____
_____

Food & Beverage

Breakfast
_____
_____

Lunch
_____
_____

Supper
_____
_____

Snacks
_____
_____

Water

Positive Things That Happened Today:

_____
_____
_____
_____
_____

Is There Anything I Could Have Done To Improve My Day:

_____
_____
_____
_____
_____

Today, I Am Grateful For:

_____
_____
_____
_____
_____

Positive Affirmations:

_____
_____
_____
_____
_____

Goals/Things I Can Do To Make Tomorrow Better:

_____
_____
_____
_____

Date: _____ Wake-Up Time For Today: _____
Hours Slept Last Night:_____

My Mood:

Morning

Afternoon   **Evening**

How I Feel Today?
- ❑ Anger/frustration
- ❑ Appetite- increased or decreased
- ❑ Difficulty concentrating/making decisions
- ❑ Energized
- ❑ Happy
- ❑ Hopeful
- ❑ Hopeless
- ❑ Joyful
- ❑ Lack of motivation
- ❑ No energy fatigue/lethargic
- ❑ Sad and/or tearful
- ❑ _____
- ❑ _____
- ❑ _____
- ❑ _____

Exercise
_____
_____
_____
_____

Food & Beverage

Breakfast
_____
_____

Lunch
_____
_____

Supper
_____
_____

Snacks
_____
_____

Water

Positive Things That Happened Today:

_____
_____
_____
_____
_____

Is There Anything I Could Have Done To Improve My Day:

_____
_____
_____
_____
_____

Today, I Am Grateful For:

_____
_____
_____
_____
_____

Positive Affirmations:

_____
_____
_____
_____
_____

Goals/Things I Can Do To Make Tomorrow Better:

_____
_____
_____
_____
_____

Date: _____ Wake-Up Time For Today: _____
Hours Slept Last Night: _____

My Mood:

Morning

Afternoon   **Evening**

How I Feel Today?
- ❏ Anger/frustration
- ❏ Appetite- increased or decreased
- ❏ Difficulty concentrating/making decisions
- ❏ Energized
- ❏ Happy
- ❏ Hopeful
- ❏ Hopeless
- ❏ Joyful
- ❏ Lack of motivation
- ❏ No energy fatigue/lethargic
- ❏ Sad and/or tearful
- ❏ _____
- ❏ _____
- ❏ _____
- ❏ _____

Exercise
_____
_____
_____
_____

Food & Beverage

Breakfast
_____
_____

Lunch
_____
_____

Supper
_____
_____

Snacks
_____
_____

Water

Positive Things That Happened Today:

_____
_____
_____
_____
_____

Is There Anything I Could Have Done To Improve My Day:

_____
_____
_____
_____
_____

Today, I Am Grateful For:

_____
_____
_____
_____
_____

Positive Affirmations:

_____
_____
_____
_____
_____

Goals/Things I Can Do To Make Tomorrow Better:

_____
_____
_____
_____
_____

Date: _____ Wake-Up Time For Today: _____

Hours Slept Last Night:_____

My Mood:

Morning

Afternoon

Evening

How I Feel Today?

- ❏ Anger/frustration
- ❏ Appetite- increased or decreased
- ❏ Difficulty concentrating/making decisions
- ❏ Energized
- ❏ Happy
- ❏ Hopeful
- ❏ Hopeless
- ❏ Joyful
- ❏ Lack of motivation
- ❏ No energy fatigue/lethargic
- ❏ Sad and/or tearful
- ❏ _____
- ❏ _____
- ❏ _____
- ❏ _____

Exercise
_____
_____
_____
_____

Food & Beverage

Breakfast
_____
_____

Lunch
_____
_____

Supper
_____
_____

Snacks
_____
_____

Water

Positive Things That Happened Today:

_____
_____
_____
_____
_____

Is There Anything I Could Have Done To Improve My Day:

_____
_____
_____
_____
_____

Today, I Am Grateful For:

_____
_____
_____
_____
_____

Positive Affirmations:

_____
_____
_____
_____
_____

Goals/Things I Can Do To Make Tomorrow Better:

_____
_____
_____
_____
_____

Date: _____ Wake-Up Time For Today: _____

Hours Slept Last Night: _____

My Mood:

Morning

Afternoon   **Evening**

How I Feel Today?

- ❑ Anger/frustration
- ❑ Appetite- increased or decreased
- ❑ Difficulty concentrating/making decisions
- ❑ Energized
- ❑ Happy
- ❑ Hopeful
- ❑ Hopeless
- ❑ Joyful
- ❑ Lack of motivation
- ❑ No energy fatigue/lethargic
- ❑ Sad and/or tearful
- ❑ _____
- ❑ _____
- ❑ _____
- ❑ _____

Exercise
_____
_____
_____
_____

Food & Beverage

Breakfast
_____
_____

Lunch
_____
_____

Supper
_____
_____

Snacks
_____
_____

Water

Positive Things That Happened Today:

_____
_____
_____
_____

Is There Anything I Could Have Done To Improve My Day:

_____
_____
_____
_____

Today, I Am Grateful For:

_____
_____
_____
_____

Positive Affirmations:

_____
_____
_____
_____

Goals/Things I Can Do To Make Tomorrow Better:

_____
_____
_____
_____

Date: _____ Wake-Up Time For Today: _____

Hours Slept Last Night: _____

My Mood:

Morning

Afternoon

Evening

How I Feel Today?
- ❏ Anger/frustration
- ❏ Appetite- increased or decreased
- ❏ Difficulty concentrating/making decisions
- ❏ Energized
- ❏ Happy
- ❏ Hopeful
- ❏ Hopeless
- ❏ Joyful
- ❏ Lack of motivation
- ❏ No energy fatigue/lethargic
- ❏ Sad and/or tearful
- ❏ _____
- ❏ _____
- ❏ _____
- ❏ _____

Exercise
_____
_____
_____
_____

Food & Beverage

Breakfast
_____
_____

Lunch
_____
_____

Supper
_____
_____

Snacks
_____
_____

Water

Positive Things That Happened Today:

_____
_____
_____
_____
_____

Is There Anything I Could Have Done To Improve My Day:

_____
_____
_____
_____
_____

Today, I Am Grateful For:

_____
_____
_____
_____
_____

Positive Affirmations:

_____
_____
_____
_____
_____

Goals/Things I Can Do To Make Tomorrow Better:

_____
_____
_____
_____

Date: _____ Wake-Up Time For Today: _____
Hours Slept Last Night:_____

My Mood:

Morning

Afternoon   **Evening**

How I Feel Today?
- ❏ Anger/frustration
- ❏ Appetite- increased or decreased
- ❏ Difficulty concentrating/making decisions
- ❏ Energized
- ❏ Happy
- ❏ Hopeful
- ❏ Hopeless
- ❏ Joyful
- ❏ Lack of motivation
- ❏ No energy fatigue/lethargic
- ❏ Sad and/or tearful
- ❏ _____
- ❏ _____
- ❏ _____
- ❏ _____

Exercise
_____
_____
_____
_____

Food & Beverage

Breakfast
_____
_____

Lunch
_____
_____

Supper
_____
_____

Snacks
_____
_____

Water

Positive Things That Happened Today:

_____
_____
_____
_____
_____

Is There Anything I Could Have Done To Improve My Day:

_____
_____
_____
_____
_____

Today, I Am Grateful For:

_____
_____
_____
_____
_____

Positive Affirmations:

_____
_____
_____
_____
_____

Goals/Things I Can Do To Make Tomorrow Better:

_____
_____
_____
_____

MY APPOINTMENTS

Date	Time	Doctor	Address

MY APPOINTMENTS

Date	Time	Doctor	Address

MY APPOINTMENTS

Date	Time	Doctor	Address

MY APPOINTMENTS

Date	Time	Doctor	Address

MY APPOINTMENTS

Date	Time	Doctor	Address

www.ingramcontent.com/pod-product-compliance
Lightning Source LLC
Chambersburg PA
CBHW081154070526
44583CB00021B/2834